YOUR KNOWLEDGE HAS VALUE

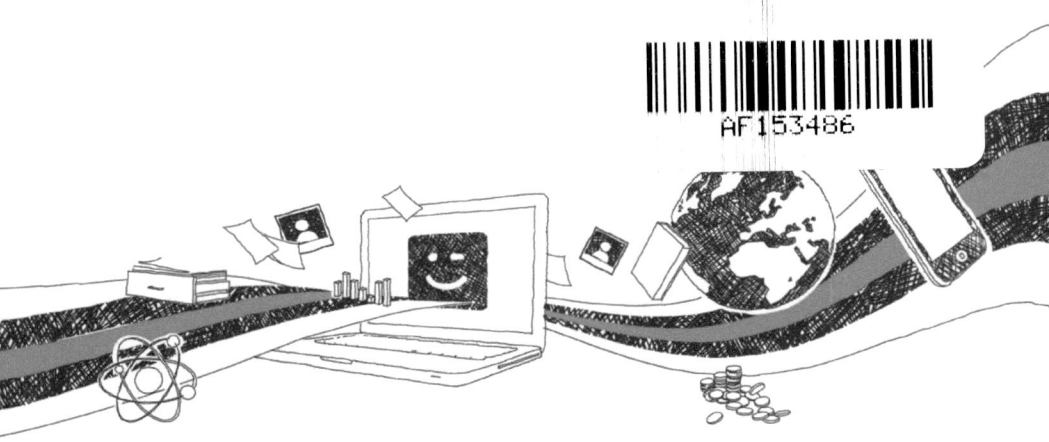

AF153486

- We will publish your bachelor's and
  master's thesis, essays and papers

- Your own eBook and book -
  sold worldwide in all relevant shops

- Earn money with each sale

Upload your text at www.GRIN.com
and publish for free

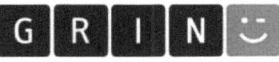

New antibiotics against pathogens

Anas Bagonaid

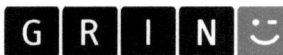

Bibliographic information published by the German National Library:

The German National Library lists this publication in the National Bibliography; detailed bibliographic data are available on the Internet at http://dnb.dnb.de.

ISBN: 9783346441393
This book is also available as an ebook.

© GRIN Publishing GmbH
Nymphenburger Straße 86
80636 München

All rights reserved

Print and binding: Books on Demand GmbH, Norderstedt, Germany
Printed on acid-free paper from responsible sources.

The present work has been carefully prepared. Nevertheless, authors and publishers do not incur liability for the correctness of information, notes, links and advice as well as any printing errors.

GRIN web shop: https://www.grin.com/document/1034840

Anhalt University of Applied Sciences

Department of Applied Biosciences and
Process Engineering

New Antibiotics

From: Anas Bagonaid

Study programme: Pharmaceutical Engineering (M.Sc.)

Table of contents

List of Abbreviations.. II

List of Figures II

1. Introduction 1

2. Antibiotics newly approved on the market since 2019 2

    2.1. Imipenem, Cilastatin and Relebactam (Recarbrio)... 4

    2.2. Pretomanid 4

    2.3. Delafloxacin... 5

    2.4. Cefiderocol 5

    2.5. Lefamulin... 5

3. New antibiotics against pathogens 6

    3.1. Challenges in the development of new antibiotics 7

    3.2. Antibiotics in the pipeline of the pharmaceutical industry 8

4. Discussion and summary 10

References 11

Appendix 13

List of Abbreviations

ABS	-	Antibiotic Stewardship
API	-	Active Pharmaceutical Ingredient
ATP	-	Adenosine Triphosphate
DNA	-	Deoxyribonucleic Acid
EMA	-	European Medicines Agency
i.v.	-	Intravenous Injection (administered into, a vein or veins)
MDR	-	Multiple Drug Resistance
MRSA	-	Methicillin-resistant Staphylococcus aureus (MRSA Super bug)
TB	-	Tuberculosis
USA	-	United States of America
USFDA	-	United States Food and Drug Administration
vfa	-	Verband forschender Arzneimittelhersteller (Association of Research-Based Pharmaceutical Companies)
WHO	-	World Health Organization

List of Figures

Number and Inscription	Page number
Fig. 1: Industrial pharmaceutical researchers in Germany, Austria and Switzerland [14]...6	
Fig. 2: The geographical distribution of the 145 facilities with Preclinical pipeline projects [18]...8	
Fig. 3: Pathogens targeted by a single pathogen-product targets [18]...9	

1. Introduction

Antibiotics are active substances that inhibit the growth of bacteria or kill them. They are administered for the treatment and also for the prevention of bacterial infectious diseases. Their effects are based on selective interaction with molecular structures that are specific to the pathogens [1].

Since their discovery over 70 years ago, antibiotics have been our most important weapon in the treatment of bacterial infections, including life-threatening hospital infections. However, they are often routinely prescribed and taken, not infrequently in an inappropriate manner. Antibiotics are also used in livestock for treatment, disease prevention and growth promotion. But their effectiveness is at risk, as antibiotic resistance has emerged through their indiscriminate use.

Antibiotic resistance is an expected natural mechanism that occurs where an antibiotic that would normally inhibit the growth of a particular bacterial or fungal species becomes weak or ineffective. Resistance to antibiotics usually occurs in combination or as an adaptation to extreme environmental conditions. According to the WHO, about 700,000 people worldwide die each year as a result of antibiotic resistance; in Germany, about 6,000 [2]. The increasing spread of resistant germs makes the development of new antibiotics urgently necessary.

Still, there is a great need for new antibiotics, especially antibiotics against multi-resistant Gram-negative bacteria in hospitals. There is also a growing need for new antibiotics against community-acquired pathogens, including those causing tuberculosis, gonorrhoea and urinary tract infections. Unless antibacterial development is revived, there is a serious risk that a growing proportion of infections, particularly in hospitals, will become effectively untreatable [3].

2. Antibiotics newly approved on the market since 2019

Despite continued efforts, physicians worldwide are constantly confronted with the threat of bacterial resistance [4]. The public health burden contributed to the development and implementation of strategies to rationally use antibiotics and limit the spread of resistant bacteria; so-called "Antibiotic Stewardship" (ABS) [5].

Another strategy in this direction is to optimise the existing pharmaceutical arsenal through novel combinations and new indications. However, the number and efficacy of these drugs are far from covering all existing needs and fully combating the highly adaptive bacterial microorganisms. Moreover, the emergence of multi-drug resistant bacteria (MDR) has already been described.

Antibiotic stewardship has proven its effectiveness, but it has its own limitations and challenges [6]. However, the search for new efficient drugs must continue and remains a pillar of the strategy against multi-resistant germs.

A number of new antibiotics and vaccines against bacterial infections are currently approved worldwide - mainly in the USA and Europe, especially Germany. An overview of the novel antibacterial agents approved by the US Food and Drug Administration (USFDA) and the European Medicines Agency (EMA) two years ago (2019) is shown in the table below (see Table 1).

Table 1: Newly approved antibiotics since 2019 [7, 8].

Active substance / mode of application	Class	Company	Areas of application	Development status
Imipenem, cilastatin and relebactam (Recarbrio), i.v.	Carbapenem, dehydropeptidase I inhibitor (booster) and beta-lactamase inhibitor	Merck & Co. (USA)	Abdominal infections, urinary tract infection and gram-negative bacteria	Approved in the EU since 02/2020, but not yet marketed; approved in the US since 07/2019 for complicated urinary tract and complicated intra-abdominal infections.
Pretomanid (for combination with bedaquiline and linezolid), oral	Nitroimidazooxazine	TB Alliance (USA & South Africa) with commercialisation partner Mylan (Netherlands)	Multidrug-resistant tuberculosis affecting the lungs	Recommended for approval in the EU since 03/2020; approved in the USA since 08/2019
Delafloxacin, i.v. / oral	Fluoroquinolone	Melinta Therapeutics (USA) and Menarini (Italy)	Skin infections, pneumonia, abdominal infections, urinary tract infection, gonorrhoea and MRSA[1]	Approved in the EU since 12/2019, but not yet marketed, approved in the USA since 06/2017
Cefiderocol, i.v.	Cephalosporin	Shionogi & Co. (Japan)	Gram-negative bacteria with limited treatment options, including Acinetobacter, Enterobacteriaceae, Pseudomonas	Approved in the EU since 04/2020; approved in the USA since 11/2019
Lefamulin, i.v. and oral	Pleuromutilin	Nabriva Therapeutics (Ireland)	Urinary tract infection, pneumonia and gram-negative bacteria	in the EU approval procedure since 06/2019; approved in the USA since 08/2019

[1] Methicillin-resistant Staphylococcus aureus (MRSA Super bug)

3

2.1. Imipenem, Cilastatin and Relebactam (Recarbrio)

Recarbrio is an antibiotic used to treat adults with infections caused by bacteria classified as aerobic gram-negative bacteria. This medicine is used when other treatments may not work. Recarbrio contains the active ingredients *imipenem*, *cilastatin* and *relebactam* [8]. This medicine is administered as an intravenous infusion.

One of the active ingredients in Recarbrio, *imipenem*, kills bacteria, while the other two, *cilastatin* and *relebactam*, increase imipenem's effectiveness in different ways. *Imipenem* interferes with bacterial proteins that are important for building the bacterial cell wall. This leads to defective cell walls that collapse and cause the bacteria to die. Imipenem is rapidly broken down by the kidneys and the *cilastatin* in Recarbrio prevents this breakdown and makes *imipenem* last longer. The third active ingredient, *relebactam*, blocks enzymes in the bacteria called beta-lactamases. These enzymes break down antibiotics like *imipenem* and stop them from working.

2.2. Pretomanid

Pretomanid is a *nitroimidazole*. In pharmacology, *nitroimidazoles* are groups of substances used to treat infections with bacteria and / or protozoa and whose core feature is an *imidazole* substituted with a nitro group. It was approved by the USFDA in August 2019 for use in combination with the active ingredients *bedaquiline* and *linezolid* [10]. This medicine is administered in the form of tablets for oral administration.

Bedaquiline has antimycobacterial properties against dividing and non-dividing tuberculosis bacteria (TB). The effects are based on the inhibition of mycobacterial ATP synthase, which is important for energy production. This prevents the formation of the energy carrier ATP. Likewise, linezolid has antibacterial properties against aerobic gram-positive bacteria, some gram-negative and anaerobic microorganisms. The effects are based on the inhibition of protein synthesis by binding to bacterial ribosomes. Unlike other antibiotics, it is effective at the beginning of translation and inhibits the formation of the initiation complex [10].

2.3. Delafloxacin

Delafloxacin is a bactericidal antibiotic from the group of *fluoroquinolones* (subgroup of quinolone antibiotics) and is mainly used for the treatment of bacterial skin infections. The effects are based on the inhibition of bacterial topoisomerase IV and DNA gyrase [11]. The drug is administered as an intravenous infusion and in the form of tablets for ingestion. Delafloxacin is predominantly glucuronidated and is hardly subject to oxidative metabolism.

2.4. Cefiderocol

Cefiderocol is an antibiotic used in adults to treat infections caused by bacteria classified as aerobic gram-negative bacteria. This medicine is administered as an intravenous infusion.

The active substance cefiderocol belongs to the class of *cephalosporin* antibiotics. Cephalosporins form a group of broad-spectrum antibiotics and, like penicillin, belong to the β-lactam antibiotics. It uses the bacteria's own system to import iron, which succeeds in the bacterial cell. Thus, the formation of the bacterial cell wall is blocked and the bacteria are killed [12].

2.5. Lefamulin

Lefamulin is a semi-synthetic antibiotic. According to the manufacturer, lefamulin is the first systemically active antibiotic for human medicine from the group of *pleuromutilins*. Pleuromutilins are a group of natural substances that originate from fungi. They inhibit protein synthesis by binding to the peptidyl transferase centre of the 50S subunit of ribosomes [13]. Since the binding site is different from the other ribosomal interacting antibacterial substances, lefamulin is said to be effective even if resistance has already developed. The drug is administered as an intravenous infusion and orally in the form of tablets.

3. New antibiotics against pathogens

The discovery of the first antibiotic, penicillin, over 90 years ago revolutionised modern medicine. Since then, antibiotics have become one of the most commonly used classes of drugs. They are used to prevent and treat infections and enable complex operations that have become routine. However, antibiotics are no longer as effective as they once were. Over time, certain bacteria, known as "superbugs", have adapted and learned to resist the effects of the drugs designed to kill them. The collective, overuse of antibiotics in humans, animals and plants has accelerated this process.

Drug-resistant infections are a serious threat to people's health today. Hundreds of thousands of people die every year from infections that can no longer be treated with existing drugs [2]. Research into new antibiotics capable of killing drug-resistant bacteria is crucial to saving modern medicine.

Currently, only a handful of large and more than fifty small and medium-sized companies worldwide are working on new antibiotics and other antibacterial drugs. Most of these operate their laboratories in the USA, but industrial pharmaceutical researchers are also working on new agents in Germany, Austria and Switzerland. This is shown in the following figure (see Figure 1) [14].

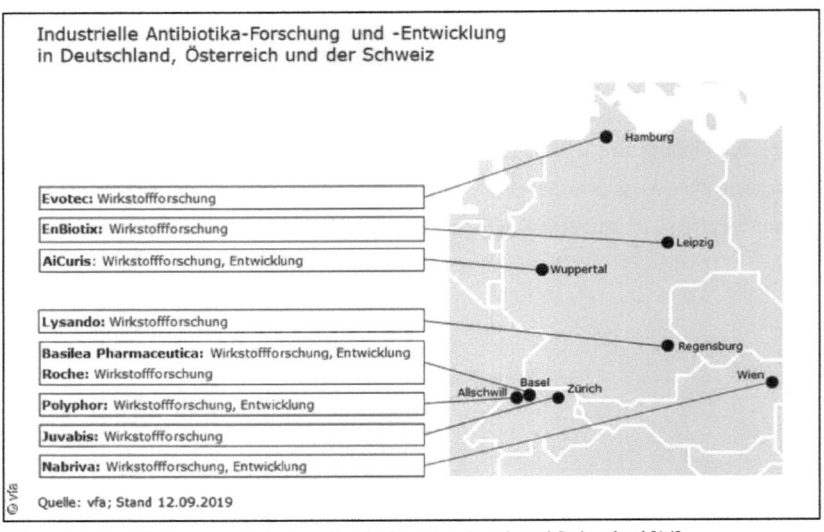

Figure 1: Industrial pharmaceutical researchers in Germany, Austria and Switzerland [14].

The figure shows that four pharmaceutical companies in Germany are researching new antibiotics. Compared to the US pharmaceutical companies (27 companies), the number is relatively small and manageable.

3.1. Challenges in the development of new antibiotics

No new classes of antibiotics have been discovered since the 1980s. A class defines a group of antibiotics that have a specific mode of action, for example by killing bacteria or stopping their multiplication, and are effective against certain types of infections [15]. The antibiotics that have been brought to market in the last three decades are variations of drugs that have been discovered previously.

The discovery and development of "novel antibiotics" or new antibiotics is a challenge. The science behind it is difficult and the research and development process is time-consuming, expensive and often fails. The development of a new antibiotic can take 10 to 15 years and cost over 1 billion US dollars [16].

Although the increasing spread of resistant germs makes the development of new antibiotics urgently necessary, the big pharmaceutical companies in particular are withdrawing more and more from this field of business. Especially when the pharmaceutical companies invest a lot of money to bring a new antibiotic to the market, but can neither cover their costs nor make a profit [15].

New antibiotics are considered "drugs of last resort" against dangerous bacteria. To limit the development of antibiotic resistance, they must be used sparingly and not sold in large quantities. In addition, antibiotics tend to be quite cheap compared to more expensive treatments. The combination of low sales and low prices limits the amount of money companies can make. Without financial incentives, many large pharmaceutical companies have begun to withdraw from research [16].

3.2. Antibiotics in the pipeline of the pharmaceutical industry

Nevertheless, according to the World Health Organization, there are currently between forty and fifty antibiotics in Phase II or III clinical trials worldwide [17]. These agents are listed in Appendix 1 (A1) of this paper.

The preclinical pipeline includes more innovative and diverse candidates - 252 antimicrobial agents are in early testing [18]. However, it will take up to ten years for the first of these drugs to reach the market. These investigated compounds are globally distributed across 145 institutions and companies (see Figure 2).

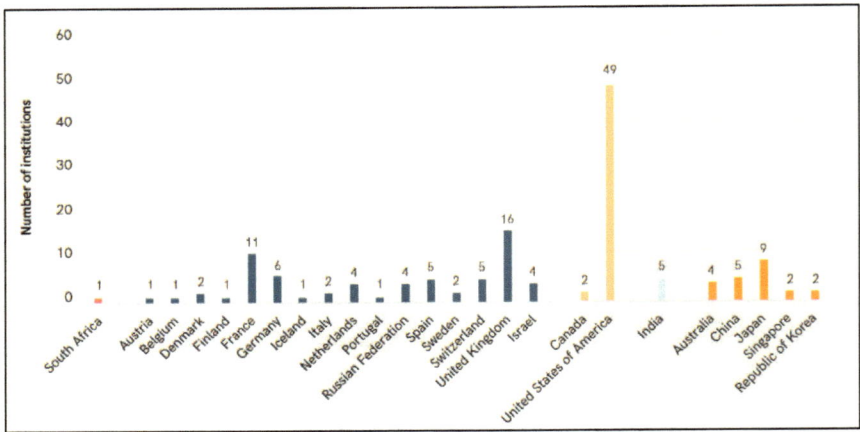

Figure 2: The geographical distribution of the 145 facilities with preclinical pipeline projects [18].

The World Health Organization's 2017 Pathogen Priority List [19] identified pathogens that cause antibiotic-resistant infections for which new antibacterial treatments are urgently needed worldwide. Examination of preclinical pipeline projects shows that a significant number of products have focused on single pathogens, representing a strong shift towards pathogen-focused therapies rather than broader-spectrum agents that can also be used empirically.

In total, 43 antibiotics target M. tuberculosis, and a further 38 antibiotics target the World Health Organization's critical Gram-negative priority pathogens (see Figure 3).

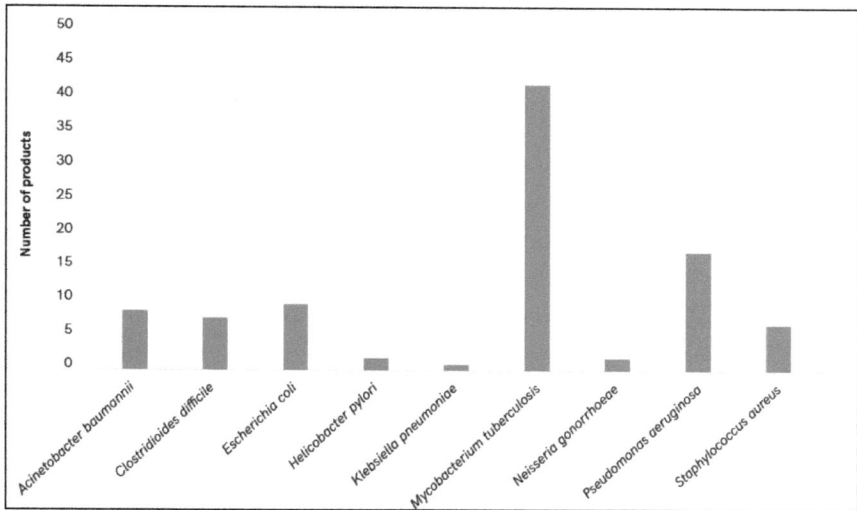

Figure 3: Pathogens targeted by a single pathogen target [18].

The main focus of the current preclinical pipeline is on Gram-negative pathogens in combination with a shift towards pathogen-specific agents. This shift likely reflects the influence of the WHO Pathogen Priority List, which highlighted resistant Gram-negatives as the most critical priority. It seems that this list has been interpreted as a guideline for companies to focus on individual pathogens rather than general bacterial infections.

4. Discussion and summary

Research into new active substances is being carried out worldwide. According to estimates by the German Association of Research-Based Pharmaceutical Companies (vfa), the pipeline is " properly" filled [14]. However, the number of these drugs that have not yet been tested on humans and will eventually reach the market is unknown.

In terms of drug development and research, the preclinical antibacterial pipeline is driven by small and medium-sized companies and academic institutions. As these companies and institutions generally rely on external funding and development partnerships, the current market dynamics and investment in antibiotic research and development do not provide a supportive environment to advance successful products beyond clinical phase I. This means that the main burden of costly research is left to medium-sized and smaller companies.

The diverse preclinical pipeline has been influenced by recent efforts to stimulate research into the development of new antibacterial agents. It is encouraging to see the different approaches being pursued in different regions of the world. As with new innovative approaches in general, most projects are likely to fail before they reach the final clinical phase. The size of the preclinical pipeline is therefore still unlikely to be sufficient to generate the much-needed innovative therapeutics. It is important to continue to invest in the discovery and preclinical phases to find and advance new antibacterial drugs to address the challenge regarding drug-resistant bacterial infections.

References

[1] Norbert Ostendorf, MD; Frank Antwerpes, MD (2018): Antibiotic - DocCheck Flexikon. DocCheck Medical Services GmbH. Available online at https://flexikon.doccheck.com/de/Antibiotikum, last updated 05.10.2018, last verified 29.05.2020.

[2] Der Spiegel (2015): Antibiotic promotes emergence of multi-resistant germs according to WHO survey - DER SPIEGEL - Gesundheit. Available online at https://www.spiegel.de/gesundheit/diagnose/multiresistente-keime-who-umfrage-enthuellte-wissensluecken-a-1063008.html, last updated 16.11.2015, last verified 29.05.2020.

[3] Livermore, D. M. (2004): The need for new antibiotics. In: Clinical microbiology and infection: the official publication of the European Society of Clinical Microbiology and Infectious Diseases 10 Suppl 4, pp. 1-9. DOI: 10.1111/j.1465-0691.2004.1004.x.

[4] Droz, Nina; Hsia, Yingfen; Ellis, Sally; Dramowski, Angela; Sharland, Mike; Basmaci, Romain (2019): Bacterial pathogens and resistance causing community acquired paediatric bloodstream infections in low- and middle-income countries: a systematic review and meta-analysis. In: Antimicrobial Resistance and Infection Control 8, p. 207. DOI: 10.1186/s13756-019-0673-5.

[5] Bretonnière, Cédric; Leone, Marc; Milési, Christophe; Allaouchiche, Bernard; Armand-Lefevre, Laurence; Baldesi, Olivier et al. (2015): Strategies to reduce curative antibiotic therapy in intensive care units (adult and paediatric). In: Intensive care medicine 41 (7), pp. 1181-1196. DOI: 10.1007/s00134-015-3853-7.

[6] Lemmen, S. W.; Lewalter, K. (2018): Antibiotic stewardship and horizontal infection control are more effective than screening, isolation and eradication. In: Infection 46 (5), pp. 581-590. DOI: 10.1007/s15010-018-1137-1.

[7] Development of new antibiotics & vaccines | vfa (2020). Available online at https://www.vfa.de/de/arzneimittel-forschung/woran-wir-forschen/antibakterielle-pipeline.html, last updated 30.04.2020, last verified 29.05.2020.

[8] Andrei, Stefan; Droc, Gabriela; Stefan, Gabriel (2019): FDA approved antibacterial drugs: 2018-2019. In: Discoveries 7 (4), e102. DOI: 10.15190/d.2019.15.

[9] Recarbrio | European Medicines Agency (2020). Available online at https://www.ema.europa.eu/en/medicines/human/EPAR/recarbrio, last updated 26.02.2020, last verified 29.05.2020.

[10] Celine Müller, Pharmacist Editor DAZ.online (2019): Pretomanid bei hochresistenter Tuberkulose. DAZ.online. Available online at https://www.deutsche-apotheker-zeitung.de/news/artikel/2019/08/20/pretomanid-bei-hochresistenter-tuberkulose, last updated 20 Aug. 2019, last verified 29.05.2020.

[11] Jorgensen, Sarah C. J.; Mercuro, Nicholas J.; Davis, Susan L.; Rybak, Michael J. (2018): Delafloxacin: Place in Therapy and Review of Microbiologic, Clinical and Pharmacologic Properties. In: Infectious Diseases and Therapy 7 (2), pp. 197-217. DOI: 10.1007/s40121-018-0198-x.

[12] Fetcroja | European Medicines Agency (2020). Available online at https://www.ema.europa.eu/en/medicines/human/EPAR/fetcroja, last updated 04.05.2020, last verified 29.05.2020.

[13] Veve, Michael P.; Wagner, Jamie L. (2018): Lefamulin: Review of a Promising Novel Pleuromutilin Antibiotic. In: Pharmacotherapy 38 (9), pp. 935-946. DOI: 10.1002/phar.2166.

[14] Antibiotics & Resistances - Securing a Head Start | vfa (2020). Available online at https://www.vfa.de/de/arzneimittel-forschung/woran-wir-forschen/neue-antibiotika-den-vorsprung-wahren.html, last updated 29.04.2020, last verified 29.05.2020.

[15] Antibiotic resistances: Pharmaceutical companies withdraw from research - WELT (2020). Available online at https://www.welt.de/wirtschaft/article205207221/Antibiotika-Resistenzen-Pharmakonzerne-ziehen-sich-aus-Forschung-zurueck.html, last updated 22.01.2020, last verified 29.05.2020.

[16] Why is it so hard to develop new antibiotics? | Wellcome (2020). Available online at https://wellcome.ac.uk/news/why-is-it-so-hard-develop-new-antibiotics, last updated 10.06.2020 last verified 29.05.2020.

[17] World Health Organization (2019): 2019 antibacterial agents in clinical development: an analysis of the antibacterial clinical development pipeline: World Health Organization.

[18] World Health Organization (2019): ANTIBACTERIAL AGENTS INPRECLINICAL DEVELOPMENT an open access database: World Health Organization.

[19] World Health Organization (2017): global priority list of antibiotic-resistant bacteria to guide research, discovery, and development of new antibiotics: World Health Organization.

Appendix

A1: New antibiotics and vaccines against bacteria in development[1]

---

[1]Development of new antibiotics & vaccines | vfa (2020). Available online at https://www.vfa.de/de/arzneimittel-forschung/woran-wir-forschen/antibakterielle-pipeline.html, last updated 30.04.2020, last verified 29.05.2020.

A1 New antibiotics and vaccines against bacteria in development

Non-pathogen-specific antibiotics with new active substance in clinical development from phase II, in the approval process or before market launch (as of 06/2020)

Abbreviations indicate the areas of application: Gram(–) = Gram-negative bacteria, Gram(+) = Gram-positive bacteria; B = abdominal infections, H = skin infections, K = bone infections, L = pneumonia, M = middle ear infection, U = urinary tract infection, W = soft tissue infections.

Active substance of the new antibiotic, application	Class	Company	Areas of application	WHO priority (see [19])	Development status
Eravacycline, i.v./oral	Tetracycline	Tetraphase	B, U incl. multiresist. gram (–), Enterobacteriaceae	WHO 1	Approved in the EU since 09/2018, but not yet marketed
Meropenem + vaborbactam, i.v.	Carbapenem + beta-lactamase inhibitor	Menarini	U, gram (–), also with certain beta-lactamase resistances, including Enterobacteriaceae	WHO 1	Approved in the EU since 11/2018, but not yet marketed (USA: approved since 08/2017 for urinary tract infections).
Delafloxacin, i.v./oral	Fluoroquinolone	Melinta Therapeutics and Menarini	H, L, B, U incl. gonorrhoea; incl. MRSA	WHO 2	Approved in the EU since 12/2019, but not yet marketed (USA: approved since 06/2017)
Imipenem + Cilastatin + Relebactam	Carbapenem + booster + new beta-lactamase inhibitor	MSD	B, U; gram (–)	WHO 1	Approved in the EU since 02/2020, but not yet marketed (USA: approved since 07/2019 for complicated urinary tract and complicated intra-abdominal infections).
Cefiderocol, i.v.	Cephalosporin	Shionogi	gram (–) with limited treatment options, including Acinetobacter, Enterobacteriaceae, Pseudomonas	WHO 1	approved in the EU since 23.04.2020 (USA: approved since 11/2019)

A1   Neue Antibiotika und Impfstoffe gegen Bakterien in Entwicklung

Active substance of the new antibiotic, application	Class	Company	Areas of application	WHO priority (see [19])	Development status
Lefamulin, i.v. and oral	Pleuromutilin	Nabriva Therapeutics	U, L; gram (-)	--	Recommended for approval in EU since 05/2019 (USA: approved since 08/2019)
Plazomicin	Aminoglycoside	Achaogen	U, L, sepsis, also MRSA and certain multidrug-resistant gram (-), enterobacteriaceae	WHO 1	in EU approval procedure since 10/2018 (USA: approved since 06/2018)
Solithromycin (T-4288)	Fluoroketolide	Fujiflm Toyama	Respiratory infections	--	Phase III (Japan: in the approval process since 04/2019)
eflavancin (TD 1792)	Glycopeptide cephalosporin heterodimer	Theravance Biopharma/R-Pharm	gram (+), also MRSA	WHO 2	Phase III
Contezolid (MRX-I)	Oxazolidinone	MicurRx	Gram (+), also MRSA and vancomycin-resistant enterococci	WHO 2, 3	Phase III[2]

[2] 2009 Withdrawal of an EU marketing authorization application

A1 Neue Antibiotika und Impfstoffe gegen Bakterien in Entwicklung

USA: in the approval process for the treatment of skin infections since 08/2018:

Lascufloxacin, i.v. Fluoroquinolone Kyorin L, M; Gram (+), also MRSA WHO 2 Phase III Levonadifloxacin Fluoroquinolone Wockhardt H-Phase III Pecycline Tetracycline Fogangren Bio H, L, U, A-Phase III Sulopenem, i.v. and oral Carbapenem Iterum (formerly Pfizer) U, B, also Gram (-)-Phase III Zabofloxacin Fluoroquinolone Dong Wha / IASO PharmaL, also MRSA WHO 2 Phase III.

South Korea: Approved since 03/2015:

Cefepime + enmetazobactam Cephalosporin + beta-lactamase inhibitor Allecra therapeutics Gram (-), U-Phase III Tebipenem, oral Carbapenem Spero Therapeutics U-Phase III Omadacycline Tetracycline analogue Paratek H, L; also, against multidrug-resistant Gram (-), MRSA, enterobacteria, haemophilus WHO 1, 2, 3 Phase III.

USA: Approved since 10/2018; has been in the approval process in EU at times:

Gepotidacin (GSK-2140944)Topoisomerase IV inhibitor GSKH, U, gonorrhoea phase III Cefepim + taniborbactam Carbapenem + betalactamase inhibitor (for serine and metallo-betalactamases) Venatorx complicated U; Carbapenem-resistant enterobacterales (CRE) and carbapenem-resistant Pseudomonas aeruginosa (CRPA)-phase III Afabicin (Debio-1450)FABI inhibitor DebiopharmH, K, Staphylococcal phase II Brilacidin PDE 4 inhibitor Innovation Pharmaceuticals H phase IICG-400549openCrystal GenomixH phase II Nafithromycin Macrolide Wockhardt A phase II Benapenem Carbapenem Sihuan Pharmaceutical U phase II TNP-2092RNA polymerase inhibitor, Topoisomerase II and IV inhibitor TenNor Therapeutics Gram(+), H-phase IIBOS-228 (LYS-228) Monobactam Boston Pharmaceuticals multidrug-resistant enterobacteria, B, U-phase II Finafloxacin, oral and i.v. Fluoroquinolone Mer Lion Pharma B, H, U-phase II [approved in the USA against otitis media].

Non-pathogen-specific antibiotics with new combination of proven active substances in clinical development from phase II, in the approval process or before market launch (status: 06/2020)

Abbreviations indicate the areas of application: Gram(-) = Gram-negative bacteria, Gram(+) = Gram-positive bacteria; B = abdominal infections, H = skin infections, K = bone infections, L = pneumonia, M = middle ear infection, U = urinary tract infection, W = soft tissue infections.

Active substance of the new antibiotic, application	Class	Company	Areas of application	WHO priority (see [19])	Development status
Aztreonam + avibactam (a monobactam and a beta-lactamase inhibitor), intravenous use	Monobactam + beta-lactamase inhibitor	Allergan	complicated B or H, L	WHO priority (see [19])	Phase III

A1 Neue Antibiotika und Impfstoffe gegen Bakterien in Entwicklung

Antibiotics targeted against specific bacteria and other anti-infectives with new active ingredient - in development (from phase II), in the approval process or before market launch (as of 03/2020)

Active substance of the new antibiotic, application	Class	Company	Areas of application	WHO priority (see [19])	Development status
omanide (for combination with bedaquiline and linezolid); oral	Nitroimidazooxazine	TB Alliance (with commercialisation partner Mylan)	multidrug-resistant tuberculosis	n.a.	Recommended for approval in the EU since 03/2020 (USA: approved since 08/2019)
Delpazolid; oral	Oxazolidinone	LegoChem	Tuberculosis	n.a.	Phase II
Macozinone (PBTZ-169, piperazine benzothiazinone); oral	DprE1 inhibitor	Nearmedic	Tuberculosis	n.a.	Phase II
OPC-167832; oral	DprE1 inhibitor	Otsuka	Tubeculosis	n.a.	Phase II
BTZ 043; oral	DprE1 inhibitor	Univ. Munich, HKI, DZIF (with EDCTP, Radboud Univ., BMBF)	Tuberculosis	n.a.	Phase II
Telacebec (Q203); oral	Imidazopyridinamide	Qurient	Tuberculosis	n.a.	Phase II
GSK-3036656; oral	Oxaborol	GSK	Tuberculosis	n.a.	Phase II
Aerucine (AR-105)	monoclonal antibodies	Aridis Pharmaceuticals	*Pseudomonas aeruginosa* (prevention)	WHO 1	Phase II
Sarecycline	Tetracycline	Paratec	Acne and facial rose	n.a.	Phase III
Anthrax immunoglobulin; i.v.	polyclonal serum	Emergent, BioSolutions	Anthrax infections	n.a.	Phase III
Obiltoxaximab	monoclonal antibodies	Elusys Therapeutics	Anthrax infections	n.a.	Phase III
Zoliflodacin; oral	Topoisomerase inhibitor	Entasis (with GARDP)	Gonorrhoea	WHO 2	Phase III

A1 Neue Antibiotika und Impfstoffe gegen Bakterien in Entwicklung

Active substance of the new antibiotic, application	Class	Company	Areas of application	WHO priority (see [19])	Development status
Durlobactam/Sulbactam	A, C, D-betalactamase inhibitor + cephalosporin	Entasis	*Acinetobacter baumannii*	WHO 1	Phase III
Tosatoxumab (AR-301)	monoclonal antibody	Aridis Pharmaceuticals	*Staphylococcus aureus* incl. MRSA	WHO 2	Phase III
Exebacase (CF-301)	Phage lysine	Contrafect	MRSA and VRSA	n.a.	Phase II
Ridinilazole	not stated	Summit Therapeutics	*Clostridium difficile* infections	n.a.	Phase III
OPS-2071	Quinolone	Otsuka	*Clostridium difficile* infections	n.a.	Phase II
DNV-3837	Quinoline-oxazolidinone hybrid	Deinove	*Clostridium difficile* infections	n.a.	Phase II
Medi-3902	Psl inhibitor/PcrV inhibitor	Medimmune	*Pseudomonas aeruginosa* infections	WHO 1	Phase II
N-Rephasin (SAL-200)	Phage lysine	Intron Biotechnology	MRSA, VRSA infections	WHO 2	Phase II
Suvratoxumab (Medi-4893)	Monoclonal antibody against toxin	Medimmune	MRSA infections	WHO 2	Phase II

A1 Neue Antibiotika und Impfstoffe gegen Bakterien in Entwicklung

Vaccines against bacterial infections (as of 04/2019)

Name of the vaccine project	Vaccine type	Company, Organisation	Application area	WHO priority	Development status
PF-06425090	Subunit vaccine	Pfizer	Prevention of *Clostridium difficile* infections	n.a.	Phase III
ExPeC4V	Conjugate vaccine	GlycoVaxyn / Janssen-Cilag	Prevention of extraintestinal *E. coli* of serotypes O1, O2, O6 and O25	n.a.	Phase II
Vaccine against streptococcus group B	Conjugate vaccine	GSK	Prevention of infections in newborns with group B streptococci through maternal vaccination	WHO 3	Phase II
PF-06760805	not stated	Pfizer	Prevention of infections in newborns with group B streptococci through maternal vaccination	WHO 3	Phase II
Shigella+	Conjugate vaccine	GlycoVaxyn	Prevention of Shigella infections	WHO 3	Phase II
VLA84 (IC84)	Subunit vaccine	Valneva	Prevention of *Clostridium difficile* infections	n.a.	Phase II
VPM 1002	Live vaccine, attenuated, recombinant	Serum Institute of India, Max Planck, VPM	Prevention and therapy of tuberculosis	n.a.	Phase III

A1 Neue Antibiotika und Impfstoffe gegen Bakterien in Entwicklung

Name of the vaccine project	Vaccine type	Company, Organisation	Application area	WHO priority	Development status
MIP	Whole cell vaccine	Cadila Pharma	Prevention and therapy of tuberculosis	– –	Phase III
M. vaccae	Subunit vaccine	Anhui Zhifei Longcom	Prevention of tuberculosis	– –	Phase III
M72 + AS01	Subunit vaccine	GSK, Aeras	Prevention of tuberculosis	– –	Phase II
DAR 901	Whole cell vaccine	Dartmouth University (USA), Aeras	Prevention of tuberculosis	– –	Phase II
H56:IC31	Subunit vaccine	SSI, Valneva, Aeras	Prevention of tuberculosis	– –	Phase II
H4: IC31	Subunit vaccine	Sanofi, SSI, Aeras	Prevention of tuberculosis	– –	Phase II
MTBVac	Live vaccine	Biofabri, Univ. Zagaroza, TBVI	Prevention of tuberculosis	– –	Phase II
TBFluO4L	Vaccine with vector	RIBSP	Prevention and therapy of tuberculosis	– –	Phase II
BCG Revaccination	Live vaccine	Aeras	Prevention of tuberculosis	– –	Phase II
ID93/GLASE	Subunit vaccine	IDRI/WT	Prevention of tuberculosis	– –	Phase II
RUTI	Whole cell vaccine	Archivel Farma	Prevention and therapy of tuberculosis	– –	Phase II

RIBSP: Research Institute Biological Safety Problems, Kazakhstan

IDRI: Infectious Disease Research Institute, Seattle

SSI: Statens Serum Institut, Copenhagen

VPM: Vaccine Project Management, Hanover

WT: Wellcome Trust

YOUR KNOWLEDGE HAS VALUE

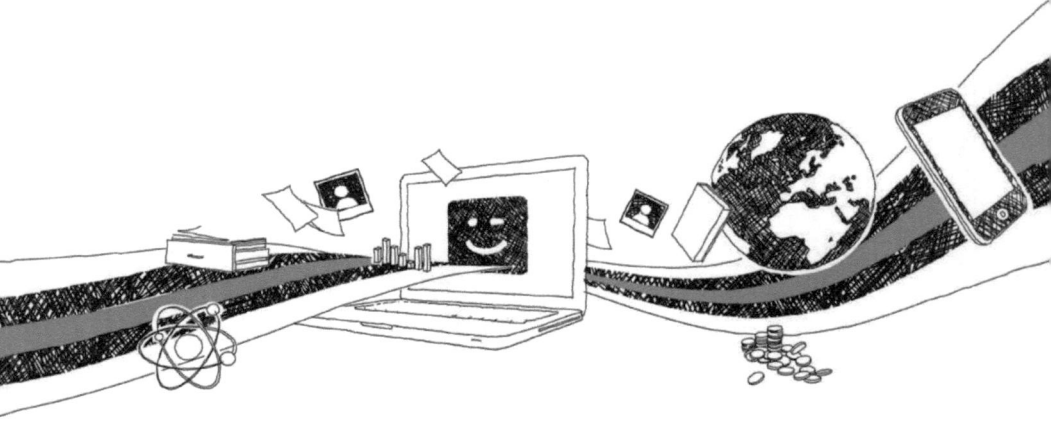

- We will publish your bachelor's and master's thesis, essays and papers

- Your own eBook and book - sold worldwide in all relevant shops

- Earn money with each sale

Upload your text at www.GRIN.com and publish for free

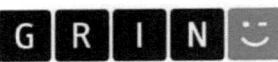